BARBARA DOREO

Ozone to Ozonoid for Rescue Dog Health

This book was professionally typeset on Reedsy.
Find out more at reedsy.com

This book is dedicated to a curly haired woman that adopted a rescue dog and within 4 months had a $10,000 veterinary bill. We now work together to share this information so that such a financial shock never happens to anyone else.

Contents

Introduction   1

What are the most common problems that a rescue
dog might...   4

What equipment will you need to work on your dog's health?   6

What other care will you need to heal your rescue dog?   11

Canine Nutrition - Things to Consider   13

Importance of Obedience Training   15

Natural Medicine Support for Various Ailments   17

Bodywork including massage, acupuncture and chiropractic   19

Success Stories   21

Troubleshooting home use   24

Conclusion   25

Credit to the artwork in this book   26

About the Author   28

Introduction

Bringing home a dog from a shelter is an exciting and fulfilling way to add to your family. Of course, there can be many challenges that come with a rescue pet as you may not know their full background in behavior and especially their health. Unfortunately for some, bringing a rescue pet into your home can turn into an incredibly expensive ordeal because of various health issues that may come along with them. Giving a rescue dog a safe loving home is very rewarding to an animal lover and it makes space in the shelter for another dog to come to the shelter. But at what price? The shelter will give you all the information that they have on your newly rescued dog. However, they don't always have all of the information or the resources to get it.

Thankfully, there are many ways to affordably help your pet heal and more easily integrate into your home. This book is designed to teach you the simple steps of helping your pet feel better with home ozone therapies and other natural remedies.

Ozone therapies can improve most health conditions affordably, lead to faster physical recovery, and also make a difference in your dog's mental wellbeing.

Ozone improves oxygenation of the dog's cells, which improves mitochondrial function. The mitochondria are the powerhouse of each cell - they produce ATP (cellular energy), the fuel for cellular regeneration and tissue healing.

Ozone kills the germs (bacteria, viruses, fungi, parasites) as it simultaneously creates energetic ozone/oxygen bonds to pep up the mitochondria. There are many studies on the PubMed database demonstrating this.

A few veterinarians have been injecting ozone gas for many decades into veins, under the skin and more as alternative therapies for various illnesses. But, as many have found, this can become expensive quickly. There are many ways to do daily treatments at home with inexpensive equipment and have great success.

Ozone is a naturally occurring substance that is always in our environment. It is continuously being made in the upper atmosphere, in the ocean waves crashing onto the shore, in lightning storms in the forest and even inside of our bodies. Unfortunately, there is just not enough in those areas to stimulate healing, so we need to give Mother Nature a boost!

You will see exactly how to do this in upcoming chapters.

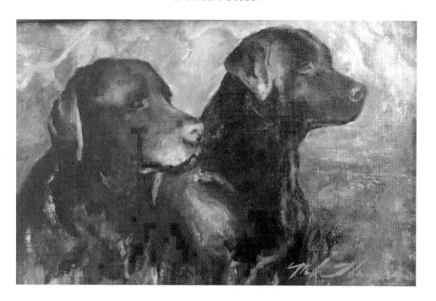

What are the most common problems that a rescue dog might have?

Fleas, Heartworms, Intestinal worms, Digestive problems, Kennel cough, Skin problems and Malnourishment are unfortunately common issues that your new pet may bring into your home.

Fleas can live up to 3 months without a host. They can live in the bedding and in furniture, which makes them a difficult pest to work with. Thankfully, ozone can be used to kill the fleas and flea eggs.

Heart worms are a serious condition. They are parasites whose larvae are carried into your dog via a mosquito bite.The heart worms travel in the dog's body to the heart and can damage the heart and lungs. Ozone can kill them too!

Intestinal worms - the five main types are roundworms, tapeworms, whipworms, and hookworms. These parasites affect each dog differently. Diarrhea and vomiting are common symptoms. Weight loss, poor coat appearance, extended belly, bright red or dark purple blood in the stool can also be signs of parasitic infection. Ozonated oil given by mouth or rectally can be helpful with this.

Digestive problems can be caused by eating spoiled food and table scraps, viral infections like parvovirus and coronavirus, bacterial infections like Campylobacteria, Salmonella, E. Coli, Clostridia, or parasites/worms. Most of these infections are spread by exposure to an infected dog's feces. Many of those infections can also be passed to humans. Ozone therapy is a powerful tool in treating these infections as it has a potent ability to destroy these organisms while helping the dog's own tissue heal faster.

Kennel cough is an upper respiratory infection most commonly caused by a bacteria called Bordetella bronchiseptica. You can treat this with ozonated oil and ozonoid gas (after bubbling ozone through oil to make it safe for the lungs).

Skin problems like allergic dermatitis, bug bites and hives cause itching, swollen eyes, red skin, diarrhea, sneezing, itchy ears, vomiting, chronic ear infections and constant licking. Ozonated water bathing, brushing with ozone gas with a hairbrush, and ozone oil applications will help.

Malnourishment can be resolved with a healthy natural foods diet. Avoid all kibble with "filler ingredients", meaning things like corn, wheat, gluten, and soy. The first few ingredients on dog food labels should be from meats and not from "meals" like "chicken meal".

What equipment will you need to work on your dog's health?

You can find small, portable, affordable air/water ozone generators online. They draw in room air which is around 20% oxygen, pass the room air through the coronal discharge tube inside where electricity interacts with the oxygen, and out comes ozone gas, O3. About 80% of what you breathe every day is nitrogen, which is relatively nonreactive, meaning it stays the same. The power is in the oxygen that goes through the machine and becomes ozone. Using room air to generate ozone is easy and quite affordable!

There are more expensive and precise ozone generators that require an oxygen tank to feed the machine. Those can produce much more concentrated and pure ozone, but that is often not necessary for home treatments. Pure and concentrated ozone is important if you were doing more invasive treatments like intravenous or blood ozone treatments.

As previously mentioned, the eyes and lungs are sensitive tissues that will get irritated with pure ozone. That means, if you have a generator running near you and you are breathing in ozone, it will make you cough and start to bother your eyes. The way to avoid this is by bubbling the ozone through organic olive or sunflower oil and then using the "ozonoid" that is produced coming out of the oil. The ozonoid is safe for all tissues.

Here are some items to have on hand to use with your ozone generator
for home therapies:
  Funnel
  Dog brush
  Plastic bags to concentrate the ozonoid gas on various body areas
  Ozonated oil
  Silicone tubing

A technique that I like to use to start working on a pet is to first brush
the dog with a brush attached to tubing from the ozone generator (an
easy way to do this is with a couple of zip-ties to hold the tubing on
the brush). I like to spray the dog's skin with ozonated water while
brushing through the fur. You can easily ozonate water by putting some
cold filtered water into a large jar or glass and putting the tube from
the ozone machine into the bottom of the glass. Let the machine run
so that the ozone bubbles into the water for at least 10 minutes, and
then your ozonated water is ready to use or drink. Note: ozone breaks
down with time, so it is recommended that ozonated water be used
within 30 minutes of making it. This technique will remove odors
and dirt without submerging the dog (which they often would like to
avoid). If you choose to submerge your dog in the bath you can use the
nanobubbler (stone on the end of ozone machine tubing) to ozonate
the bathwater before putting them in for extra sterilization.

Next, I like to put ozone oil on any breaks in the dog's skin. Ozonated
oil is also good to put on areas where the skin and fur are not growing
normally.

We then run the ozone from the generator through organic olive or sunflower oil to produce ozonoid gas (this is also how you make ozonated oil). The ozonoid gas is safe to use as it will not harm the cornea of your eyes or damage your lungs. The same is true for your dogs. After about 100 hours of bubbling, oil is fully ozonated and is ready to be used for wound care, internal and external applications. Pour your newly produced ozone oil into a 2 ounce glass bottle with an eye dropper top.

You can fill vegetable capsules with ozonated oil to use for swallowing for gut issues and parasites and they can be used as rectal suppositories.

Ozonated oil can be gently applied to the eyelids to heal eye problems and a few drops can be put in the ears for smelly, infection-prone ears.

You can brush your dog's teeth with ozonated oil to stop gingivitis, blooding gums, and bad breath. Include some flavor that your dog likes to make this job easier.

Putting ozonated oil on itchy skin helps get rid of pathogens that may be causing the itching while helping the skin heal at the same time.

Bagging is another great way to treat different areas. You can bag a sore foot, a leg, injured hind quarters, a sick belly all the way up to the neck. The trick is to use a soft, non-crinkly or noisy plastic bag to gently put over the body part to be treated with the ozone tube bringing the ozonoid gas from the oil bottle into the bag. You may want to use some string to gently tie around the limb at the top of the bag to keep the bag there. As you are setting this up and sitting with the dog, they think you are just cuddling and petting them - how easy!

Usually we do a 20 minute treatment and then the dog often will be sleepy and want to take a nap. Consider this as time for the body to heal.

Repeat your dog's ozone therapy treatments daily. Be sure to ozonate the dog's bedding too to remove irritating bugs and parasites. This can be done by putting the bedding into a large garbage bag with the ozone tube inside and letting the machine run for an hour.

Here is a picture of a common and affordable machine we have used: (Enaly OZX-300AT)

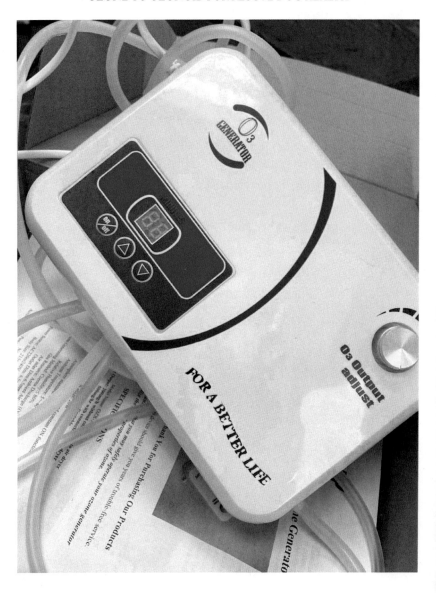

What other care will you need to heal your rescue dog?

Y ou are likely a compassionate person to even be reading this book. Showering your rescue dog with love is a good beginning. A well fitting, comfortable collar is a must. Try on different styles to see how it fits and how he/she moves in the collar. Remember, as your new rescue dog matures and fills out, their bones and muscles will take on a better shape and may need a new collar to accommodate his/her growth.

Encouraging daily exercise will be important for the dog's healing. Of course, be mindful of the pet's current abilities and be careful not to push them too hard. Daily walks are a good place to start, then you can build to fetching a ball or playing with a soccer ball for some time every day. This is also important for behavior. If a dog has too much pent up energy, they will often start acting out and chewing on things they shouldn't be.

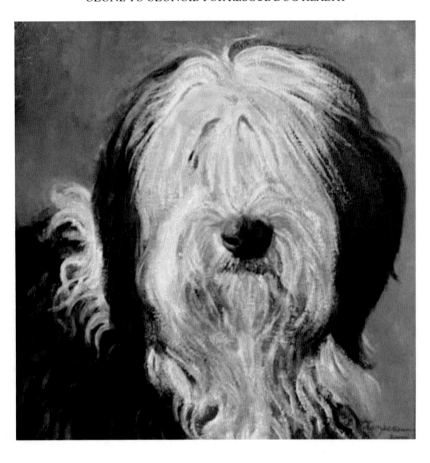

Canine Nutrition - Things to Consider

In 1970's dogs lived to 17 years old on average. Today dogs are living only about 11 years. What's the problem? Research shows that the packaged dog food from the grocery story isn't all that your dog needs. Just as with humans, if dogs are not getting the nutrients their cells need, their tissues cannot heal and regenerate.

Adequate nutrition is crucial for a strong immune system. Nutrients like vitamins C and E, zinc, and antioxidants help support a dog's immune function, helping them resist and recover from illnesses.

High-quality dog food with the right balance of fiber promotes healthy digestion. Proper digestion ensures that dogs can absorb essential nutrients from their food, preventing digestive issues such as diarrhea or constipation.

Certain nutrients like glucosamine and chondroitin contribute to joint health and can be beneficial, especially for larger breeds or senior dogs prone to arthritis and joint problems.

Nutrients like omega-3 and omega-6 fatty acids contribute to a healthy coat and skin. They can help reduce itching, inflammation, and promote a shiny, lustrous coat.

Proper nutrition can also impact a dog's behavior and cognitive function. Nutrients like essential fatty acids, antioxidants, and vitamins support brain health and may contribute to improved behavior and learning.

If you're using kibble, it should have good proteins as mentioned previously. Fruit and vegetable ingredients can also improve the dog's health and reduce the likelihood of getting cancer and other diseases. While preparing your meals you can put some bits such as chopped carrots, celery, cabbage, beets, blueberries, cherries, pumpkin and more into your dog's dish.

If your dog has any signs of allergies, it is immensely important that you improve the quality of their food, as poor food quality causes leaky gut and that often leads to developing allergies.

If the base of the dog's food is a good quality kibble, we like to have some other nutritious real food ingredients to put on top like cooked organ meats, bone broth, sardines, or sometimes even an egg. Remember, dogs are largely carnivores, so more animal proteins are healing foods for them - plus, pups love this stuff!

Importance of Obedience Training

I t's usually difficult to know how a rescue dog was treated in the past and what they have learned about certain activities, sounds, or homelife. The idea of obedience training may seem harsh for a stressed animal, but it can provide stability and other benefits, such as:

- Establishing trust: Obedience training provides a structured environment that helps build trust between the rescue dog and their new owner or handler. Positive reinforcement during training creates a positive association and strengthens the bond between the dog and their caregiver.
- Social skills: Many rescue dogs may not have had proper socialization experiences. Obedience training exposes them to different environments, people, and other animals, helping them become more comfortable and confident in various situations.
- Behavioral issues: Rescue dogs may exhibit behavioral issues such as anxiety, fear, or aggression due to past experiences. Obedience training addresses these issues by teaching alternative behaviors, building confidence, and providing a consistent and predictable routine.
- Safety: Obedience training is crucial for ensuring the safety of both the dog and the people around them. Commands like "sit," "stay," and "come" can be essential in preventing dangerous situations,

especially in public places or around other dogs and people.

- Adaptation to a new environment: Rescue dogs often need to adapt to a new home, routine, and family dynamics. Obedience training helps them understand and adjust to the rules and expectations in their new environment, reducing stress and promoting a smoother transition.

- Preventing unwanted behaviors: Training helps prevent undesirable behaviors such as excessive barking, jumping, or destructive chewing. Teaching commands and reinforcing positive behavior sets clear boundaries and expectations for the dog.

- Boosting confidence: Many rescue dogs may lack confidence due to past traumas. Obedience training provides them with a sense of accomplishment and mastery, boosting their confidence and helping them feel more secure in their new surroundings.

- Supporting communication: Obedience training establishes a communication channel between the dog and the owner. Clear communication through commands and cues helps the dog understand what is expected of them and strengthens the human-canine relationship.

It's important to approach obedience training with patience, positive reinforcement, and an understanding of the individual needs and history of each rescue dog. Consistency and a calm, supportive training environment contribute significantly to the success of training efforts. If necessary, seeking the guidance of a professional dog trainer can be beneficial in addressing specific challenges.

Natural Medicine Support for Various Ailments

H omeopathic remedies:
These are natural, non-toxic remedies that do not interfere with other medications or supplements. These remedies are easily found in most grocery or drug stores, typically in a 12C or 30C potency. These can be given right into the dog's mouth every couple of hours for acute symptoms until improvement is seen. Do not mix with food.

- Apis Mellifica: for insect bites or stings that are red and irritated
- Arnica Montana: for pain, swelling, and injuries
- Arsenicum Album: for vomiting and diarrhea, especially after eating spoiled food
- Borax (homeopathic only, not powder): for fear of loud noises like fireworks or thunderstorms
- Hepar Sulph: for infections with abscess, including infected anal glands
- Hypericum: for pain related to nerve damage/injury
- Rhus Tox: for painful/stiff arthritis and red itchy skin rashes
- Ruta Graveolens: for injuries to tendons/ligaments, especially knee or hip injuries
- Ledum Palustre; for puncture wounds and insect bites that cause

bruising

Other supplements:
If you have seen signs of digestive problems with your dog or they have had recent antibiotic use, getting a probiotic to put in their food will make a big difference.

To keep supplements simple, the pet formulas from the Standard Process brand are well-rounded to target areas of your pet's health that you may know are a problem. The powder form of those supplements are also very easy to add into their food.

When your dog's food is mostly dry, and especially when they have dry flaky skin, adding some oil to their food is a great addition. This can be any high quality fish oil or salmon oil that you would use yourself. We have also used good organic olive oil.

Bodywork including massage, acupuncture and chiropractic

Dogs love massage. Their muscles get kinked and tight just like ours, especially if they have had a stressful or traumatic past. Their joints get stiff and sore from too little exercise or after a hard day of catching Frisbees. You can follow these directions for a little massage starter.

Start at the head and use a soft, flowing gentle touch around the ears, down under the chin, back up to the neck and then around the shoulder blades. Use light to moderate pressure, depending on how your pet is responding (it should be relaxing for them). Repeat 3 to 5 times before moving onto the front legs and feet. Speaking softly, singing or humming helps your dog relax and builds trust. Next massage your dog's throat (gently), chest and stomach. You can lift and roll the skin on your dogs back to release tension. Work all the way from the head to the tail lifting and rolling the loose skin in your fingers. As you repeat this 5 times, the skin becomes looser and more flexible. Massage the hind legs by rolling them one at a time between your open hands. Start slowly and roll faster as you get to the fifth repetition. Do the same on the other leg. Stand or sit behind your dog, gently grip his hips and do an alternating rolling motion to increase hip flexibility. Lastly gently tug on your dog's tail to lengthen the spine while imbibing fluid into the disc spaces. Your Acupuncturist can recommend special points to rub to release tension. Your chiropractor can recommend special spots to massage and gently stretch to help keep your dog in his/her best posture.

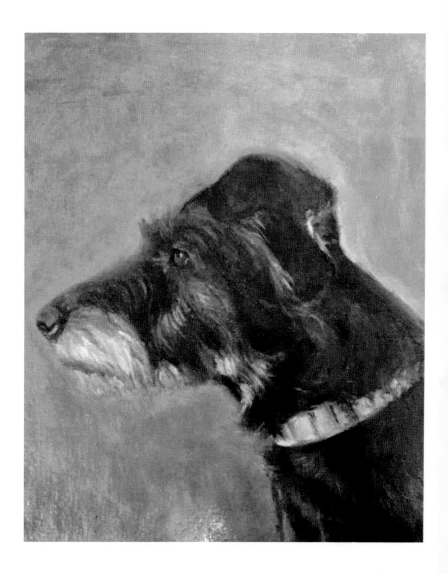

Success Stories

A sweet, cheerful, friendly young chocolate lab (CL for short) developed cancer in his nose. It was oozing and bloody. The vet recommended an expensive disfiguring surgery to remove the cancerous tissue. The owner, Janie, wanted to try ozone/ozonoid treatments first. She was diligent in performing daily treatments for CL which included Ozonoid gas through a funnel onto the nose. This was tricky at first, but CL was patient and put up with the 5 minute treatments followed by ozone oil slathered on the tumor projecting out of the nose several inches. CL drank freshly ozonated water which had run through a carbon filter. Janie drizzled 2 dropperfuls of ozonated oil on CLs food daily. This treatment continued daily for two months. The tumor shrunk. There was no more oozing or bleeding and Janie was very happy to have a clean house. CL became a happy, pain-free dog and looked like a normal-nosed chocolate lab - no surgery necessary!

Sassy was a skinny, bony, exhausted dog on the street with matted hair, and runny eyes and nose. Lisa knew she could help. She started Sassy's new life at her house with a warm ozonated water bath to loosen the matting in her hair. This was followed by the ozone hairbrush in the warm sunshine in the backyard. The ozonated water cleaned and healed Sassy's eyes and nose. Lisa discovered scabs on Sassy's skin that she applied ozone oil to by gently rubbing it into the skin. Sassy had a sore paw that Lisa also rubbed ozone oil onto. Sassy's digestion wasn't good, she clearly had a hard time doing her business. Lisa gave her small amounts of raw meat with a few vegetables and a few drops of ozone oil on top. She also had ozonated filtered water to drink. Within a few months, Lisa and Sassy were running through the neighborhood, both living a playful happy life.

A snaggle-toothed dog named Rosie had twitches and tremors. Her hind legs gave out when she tried to walk. But her sweet little Chihuahua face made you want to hug her. Ricardo carried Rosie everywhere he went. He discovered that bagging Rosie's little body with Ozonoid gas gave strength to her legs and helped calm her tremors. So, each evening after dinner, he would put her in a plastic bag in his lap with Ozonoid gas running over her. This procedure continued most evenings and Rosie continued to improve over a couple of months until she was walking easily.

A terrier named Jack had itchy ears. He put his ear to the carpet and scurried as quick as he could, then the other ear! Maxie, his new owner, held the Ozonoid gas tube near each ear for a few minutes then gently rubbed ozone oil inside his ear with her fingertips. Repeating this daily succeeded in stopping the itching in Jack's ears but he immediately started the Butt Scoots. An itchy butt needs to be treated ASAP! An ozone warm water bath to thoroughly wash the back end followed by the funnel of ozone gas over his behind, along with ozone oil gently rubbed into the anus (wear gloves for this part!) was done daily until the butt scoots stopped. Then, Jack was a happy, non-itchy guy!

Ella adopted Chloe, a 65 pound 6 month old bundle of puppy love. One year later, Chloe developed a tumor on her right front leg. Ella consulted many doctors and the diagnosis varied from "The tumor will go away if you can keep Chloe from licking it" to "I recommend that you euthanize Chloe". Ella's friend suggested she apply ozone oil to the tumor. In a couple of weeks, the tumor shrank a bit and started to heal. Ella borrowed an ozone generator to bag the leg 10 minutes 4 times a day and apply ozone oil after each ozone treatment. Ella put a collar on Chloe so she couldn't lick the healing tumor in the meantime. Ella bought a smaller ozone generator (Enaly 300 AT) but it wasn't strong enough to produce enough healing ozone to do the job so she returned that one and bought a stronger generator (A2Z 3000). Ella continued daily treatments with good results - the tumor appears to be completely resolved. This is just another affordable, noninvasive healing success story!

Troubleshooting home use

Why doesn't the oil bubble quickly when I ozonate it? The oil thickens over time as ozone bubbles through it. Some of the ozone interacts with the oil so the oil holds onto it and over a period of days it becomes thicker and stickier. When it is too thick, it's time to replace the oil and cut a small piece from the end of the tubing in the oil if it's clogged.

How do I know if the machine is making ozone?

Ozone has a very particular smell that you will notice as soon as you turn the machine on. Ozone is made in the atmosphere during a lightning storm and many say the smell is similar to the "clean" or "fresh" air smell after a storm. You will not see the ozone coming out of the machine as it is a clear gas, just like air.

In the case of accidental direct ozone inhalation that causes coughing (be careful to avoid this), immediately drink some cold water with added vitamin C to reverse potential oxidation.

Conclusion

We can use ozone therapy to penetrate the skin, get into circulation, and travel to the location that needs to heal. Ozonated water can be used for bathing and provide clean drinking water that helps to heal the digestive system.

Ozonated oil can be used to heal wounds, rashes, bites and injuries inside and out.

When the ozone gas bubbles through polyunsaturated oils, its structure changes and becomes ozonoid. Ozonoid doesn't have any negative side effects and it smells less pungent than ozone itself. It is also safe to use near eyes and lung tissue.

These simple techniques can be used by anyone at home to encourage healing. This reduces the cost of veterinary care and reduces the need for pharmaceuticals. We have seen wonderful results with these simple therapies in many cases where multiple pharmaceuticals and surgical intervention would have been standard veterinary practice. Empower yourself by learning about these techniques, as they are invaluable.

Credit to the artwork in this book

T he wonderful artwork included in these pages was created by Mark Thompson. Here is some information on him and his work:

"Painting and drawing for me, begins with beauty. A person or place, real or imagined, draws me in. This inspires me and challenges me to create my personal vision. My goal in portraiture is to capture that special look of the subject. The fundamentals aren't enough. Without passion and emotion, my work won't resonate - for me or any viewer.

Each piece is a leap of faith. The journey from inspiration to art is intuitive. That first step is uncertain. I feel my way, stroke by stroke. When things go well, I'm in the zone, focused, oblivious to time. How to begin? Where to end? There are no rules. I know it when I get there. Then I clean my palette and wait for the next beautiful inspiration.

I am a member of Ojai Studio Artists. I welcome portrait commission work, by appointment.

Contact me at MarkThompson@DSLextreme.com or www.MarkThompsonPortraitsAndFineArt.com "

CREDIT TO THE ARTWORK IN THIS BOOK

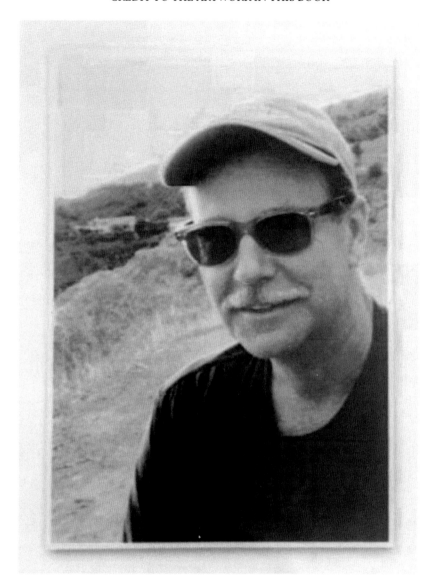

27

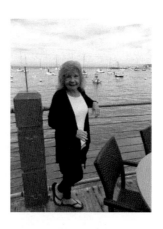

About the Author

Dr Barbara Doreo is a Chiropractor and Dental Hygienist with many years of experience in helping people improve their health. She has nurtured a family involved in natural medicine through her daughter that practices as a Chiropractor and Naturopathic Doctor, as well as her granddaughter practicing as a Naturopathic Doctor.

Dr Doreo has seen amazing healing while using the methods in this book. She believes that everyone should have access to this information and be empowered to help their loved ones live life feeling well. Her passion is in showing people simple and affordable methods to use at home to encourage healing of many different health issues, especially when conventional methods have been unsuccessful.

Made in the USA
Monee, IL
20 September 2024

65524308R00021